Student Workbook

Self-Care for New and Student Nurses

Dorrie K. Fontaine, PhD, RN, FAAN

Tim Cunningham, DrPH, MSN, RN, FAAN

Natalie May, PhD

Sigma
GLOBAL NURSING EXCELLENCE

Sigma Theta Tau International Honor Society of Nursing (Sigma) is a nonprofit organization whose mission is developing nurse leaders anywhere to improve healthcare everywhere. Founded in 1922, Sigma has more than 135,000 active members in over 100 countries and territories. Members include practicing nurses, instructors, researchers, policymakers, entrepreneurs, and others. Sigma's more than 540 chapters are located at more than 700 institutions of higher education throughout Armenia, Australia, Botswana, Brazil, Canada, Colombia, Croatia, England, Eswatini, Ghana, Hong Kong, Ireland, Israel, Italy, Jamaica, Japan, Jordan, Kenya, Lebanon, Malawi, Mexico, the Netherlands, Nigeria, Pakistan, Philippines, Portugal, Puerto Rico, Scotland, Singapore, South Africa, South Korea, Sweden, Taiwan, Tanzania, Thailand, the United States, and Wales. Learn more at www.sigmanursing.org.

Sigma Theta Tau International
550 West North Street
Indianapolis, IN, USA 46202

To request a review copy for course adoption, order additional books, buy in bulk, or purchase for corporate use, contact Sigma Marketplace at 888.654.4968 (US/Canada toll-free), +1.317.687.2256 (International), or solutions@sigmamarketplace.org.

To request author information, or for speaker or other media requests, contact Sigma Marketing at 888.634.7575 (US/Canada toll-free) or +1.317.634.8171 (International).

ISBN: 9781646480340
PDF ISBN: 9781646480371

Publisher: Dustin Sullivan
Acquisitions Editor: Emily Hatch
Development Editor: Meaghan O'Keeffe
Cover Designer: Rebecca Batchelor
Interior Design/Page Layout: Rebecca Batchelor

Managing Editor: Carla Hall
Publications Specialist: Todd Lothery
Project Editor: Meaghan O'Keeffe
Copy Editor: Gill Editorial Services
Proofreader: Jane Palmer

Table of Contents

About the Authors

Dorrie K. Fontaine, PhD, RN, FAAN (she/her), is the Dean Emerita at the University of Virginia (UVA) School of Nursing, where she served as dean for 11 years until 2019. A champion of creating healthy work environments in clinical and academic settings, she is a Past President of the American Association of Critical-Care Nurses (AACN). In 2009 she created the Compassionate Care Initiative at UVA, which has grown to be a guiding force in transforming the culture of the school with a focus on fostering human flourishing and resilience for students, faculty, and staff. A noted author of critical-care texts, a leadership book, and multiple papers and presentations on creating healthy work environments through compassionate care, Fontaine credits a spring 2009 retreat at Upaya Zen Center in Santa Fe with the Abbot Roshi Joan Halifax for setting her on the path of mindfulness, meditation, and a renewed focus on self-care. She attended Villanova University and the University of Maryland, and she received her PhD from The Catholic University of America. Her four-decade career of teaching and academic leadership includes the University of Maryland, Georgetown University, and the University of California, San Francisco (UCSF). Fontaine lives in Washington, D.C., and the Blue Ridge Mountains of Virginia with her husband, Barry.

Tim Cunningham, DrPH, MSN, RN, FAAN (he/him), began his professional career as a performing artist and clown. As a clown, he worked for two organizations that changed his life. The first, The Big Apple Circus, employed him to perform as a clown doctor at Boston Children's Hospital, Yale New Haven Children's Hospital, and Hasbro Children's Hospital. Concurrently, he volunteered for Clowns Without Borders (CWB), performing in various refugee camps, war zones, and other global zones of crisis. He later served as Executive Director of CWB. It was in pediatric hospitals and refugee camps where he witnessed and began to learn about the true meaning of resilience and self-care. This performance work inspired him to pursue a career in nursing, and he completed a second-degree nursing program at the University of Virginia. Cunningham became an emergency trauma nurse and worked clinically in Charlottesville, Virginia; Washington, D.C.; and New York City. During his time in New York City, he completed his doctoral degree in public health at the Mailman School of Public Health, Columbia University. Cunningham is the former Director of the Compassionate Care Initiative at the University of Virginia, where he had the opportunity to work closely with Drs. Fontaine and May as this book came to fruition. He currently lives in Atlanta, Georgia, and serves as the Vice President of Practice and Innovation at Emory Healthcare, where he also holds a joint appointment as an adjunct Assistant Professor at the Nell Hodgson Woodruff School of Nursing at Emory University. Cunningham began his academic journey receiving his BA in English from the College of William and Mary in 2000. For self-care, he is an avid runner and wanna-be gardener. He also loves any chance he can get to swim in the ocean or meditate as the sun rises.

Natalie May, PhD (she/her), recently transitioned to the University of Virginia (UVA) School of Nursing after 30 years as Associate Professor of Research in the Division of General Medicine, UVA School of Medicine. She is a founding member of the UVA Center for Appreciative Practice. Certified as an Appreciative Inquiry facilitator and lead author of *Appreciative Inquiry in Healthcare*, she enjoys developing Appreciative Inquiry projects and teaching appreciative practice workshops at her home institution and beyond. May is an experienced qualitative researcher, and she has extensive grant writing, program and curriculum development, and program evaluation experience. Her current research projects include the Mattering in Medicine study and the Medical Subspecialties HOME Team Program for high utilizer patients. She was also an investigator for the Wisdom in Medicine Project: Mapping the Path Through Adversity to Wisdom, a study funded by the John Templeton Foundation. She is coauthor of *Choosing Wisdom: The Path Through Adversity* and coproducer of a PBS film, *Choosing Wisdom*. She has codeveloped and implemented an innovative curriculum for medical students, The Phronesis Project, designed to foster wisdom in young physicians, and has implemented a similar program, Wisdom in Nursing, in the UVA School of Nursing. May earned a BA in economics and urban studies from Wellesley College, an MA in creative writing from Boston University, and her PhD in educational research from the University of Virginia Curry School of Education. She lives in Richmond, Virginia, with her husband, Jim. Her most consistent and effective self-care practices are modern quilting and walking near water, especially the James River and the ocean at the Outer Banks, North Carolina.

Contributing Authors

Writing this book was an exciting opportunity to collaborate with some of the people we enjoy and admire most. We reached out to our friends and colleagues in nursing and related fields to bring you diverse perspectives on self-care and to add their expertise to the conversation. In addition to nurses, we have physicians, researchers, advocates, a lawyer, a psychologist, members of the clergy, hospital administrators, and a nurse historian. We are especially pleased that so many nurses generously share their stories with you here. We have done our best to include diverse perspectives and to cast a wide net around the topic of self-care in nursing. We hope you agree that our collaborators' insights strengthen the book and offer self-care ideas that you may not find anywhere else.

We thank the following authors for their thoughtful writing on the topic of self-care for nurses. We are especially grateful to Gina DeGennaro, DNP, CNS, RN, AOCN, CNL and Edie Barbero, PhD, RN, PMHNP-BC at the University of Virginia School of Nursing for their wealth of expertise as well as their teaching insights.

Kim Acquaviva, PhD, MSW, CSE (she/her)

Ryan Bannon, BSN, RN, CCRN (he/him)

Jonathan Bartels, BSN, RN (he/him)

Susan Bauer-Wu, PhD, RN, FAAN (she/her)

Robin C. Brown-Haithco, MDiv (she/her)

Reynaldo "Ren" Capucao, Jr., MSN, RN, CNL (he/him)

Ebru Çayir, MD, PhD (she/her)

Hannah R. Crosby, BA, RYT (she/her)

Anna DeLong, LCSW, CEAP, MSW, BA (she/her)

Dallas Ducar, MSN, RN, PMHNP-BC, CNL, NREMT-B (she/her)

Lerner L. Edison, MSN, MA, RN, CNL (he/him)

Linda Grabbe, PhD, FNP-BC, PMHNP-BC, FAAN (she/her)

Valérie Gruhn, MPH, BSN, RN (she/her)

Julie Haizlip, MD, MAPP (she/her)

Susan Hassmiller, PhD, RN, FAAN (she/her)

Ashley R. Hurst, JD, MDiv, MA (she/her)

Nicole Jefferson, BSN, RN (she/her)

Master Hiromi Hangai Johnson (she/her)

Mick Krasner, MD, FACP (he/him)

Irène P. Mathieu, MD (she/her)

Michelle Maust, MD, FAPA (she/her)

Carrie McDermott, PhD, APRN, ACNS-BC (she/her)

Joy Miller, MSN, BS, RN, CPNP-PC, CPN (she/her)

K. Jane Muir, BSN, RN (she/her)

Sharon Pappas, PhD, RN, NEA-BC, FAAN (she/her)

Kate M. Pfeiffer, MS, PMHCNS-BC, PMHNP-BC (she/her)

Elizabeth A. (Lili) Powell, PhD (she/her)

Millie Sattler, DNP, MSN, RN, CCRN (she/her)

Victoria Tucker, BSN, RN (she/her)

Kath Weston, PhD (she/her)

Introduction: Building Your Self-Care Tool Kit

To ensure that we're all on the same page, let's revisit a few key points from the textbook.

- Self-care is not selfish. Nurses should be entitled, in fact expected, to care for themselves with the same creativity and compassion that they use to care for others.

- Nurses don't flourish simply by fostering the well-being of others. The nursing profession is inherently meaningful in that we care for patients and families during their most vulnerable moments. But meaningful work has its limits. A major thread throughout this book is that we don't want to be "the naked person offering someone their coat."

- Self-care is about the mind as much as it is about the body.

- Self-care is a lifelong *practice*, and it is best to begin the practice early, before facing the stressors of a hospital or other clinical setting. In general, student nurses face significantly more stress than their peers, increasing the importance and value of self-care practices during nursing school.

- Individual self-care practices do not let organizations off the hook. The importance of a healthy work environment cannot be overstated, and in this book, we offer help in selecting a healthy workplace and encourage readers to advocate for themselves and others.

Building a Self-Care Tool Kit

This workbook will provide opportunities for you, the student nurse or new graduate nurse, to explore self-care behaviors that will help you deal with the big and small stressors you will encounter in your life or that you are encountering now. Our hope for you is that you will wholeheartedly "jump in" and explore both the practices outlined in this book and others that you encounter in this journey. Self-care has become an exciting field of study and practice, especially during the time of COVID-19 and other stressors that affect those of us who work in healthcare. There are so many resources to explore, and we have designed this workbook to encourage you to take advantage of as many of them as you can.

We encourage you to build your own self-care tool kit. Just like a carpentry tool kit or any tool kit, it will contain important items to help you be the best nurse (or carpenter) possible. The tools are essential to getting the job done. This self-care tool kit, instead of hammers, screw drivers, and tape measures, will be a collection of a strategies, behaviors, and mindsets that will help you flourish in nursing.

To that end, we hope that you will try many of the practices shared here. Some will resonate with you immediately. Some will fit your lifestyle. Some will need modifying to suit your preferences. (Don't like writing down a gratitude list with paper and pen? Take photographs or use social media instead.) Some will just be completely wrong for you. Some might be intriguing to you, but maybe you'll decide to hold off and try them again in a few months or years. Explore practices on your own. If you are in a classroom or group setting, take advantage of your collective wisdom, and share your explorations with each other.

We cannot emphasize this enough: *These practices take practice!* So much of self-care is mental work, even more than the physical work of caring for your body. Our human brains are blessed with neuroplasticity, or the capacity to change. Just as you can build muscle tissue and train yourself in a physical skill such as bowling, roller skating, or playing the tuba, you can train your brain to react in new ways to stress and the challenges of your chosen profession.

When you have completed the readings in the textbook and the exercises in this workbook, we anticipate that you will have your own collection of self-care tools that you can practice regularly and rely on when you face challenges in your career and life. This self-care tool kit will help you build resilience to overcome a range of adversities, from daily annoyances, to ongoing stressors, to sudden loss or change.

The What-Why-Do-Reflect & Journal Format

The chapters in this workbook correspond to the chapters in *Self-Care for New and Student Nurses* (Fontaine, Cunningham, & May, 2021). The workbook exercises have been designed by the authors in consultation with our workbook chapter contributors. We encourage you to use the workbook as a complement to the textbook.

As nurses, we appreciate nothing more than order and structure. (Consider reporting structures, care plans, and checklists.) We take that approach with this workbook. We call it the *What-Why-Do-Reflect & Journal* format, and you will become very familiar with it as you move through this workbook. The *What-Why-Do-Reflect & Journal* structure provides a framework for exploring self-care behaviors by learning (or reviewing) what they are and why they matter for your well-being; trying them; and reflecting upon their usefulness to you in your life and clinical practice. By journaling, we encourage you to not only reflect on your progress but keep track of which techniques feel right to you, which ones might need tweaking, and which ones might serve you well in the future.

section I
Fundamentals

1

The Fundamentals of Stress, Burnout, and Self-Care

what

- Read Chapter 1.
- What do we mean by the phrase "a naked person offering someone their shirt"?
- Describe the differences between stress, stressors, and burnout.
- List five stressors that nurses face in the workplace that are unique to healthcare and nursing.
    1.
    2.
    3.
    4.
    5.
- Why are new and early-career nurses more vulnerable to burnout and stress-related ill health than more experienced nurses?
- What barriers to self-care might you face as a practicing nurse?

why

- List three reasons a personal self-care practice is important for nurses.

    1.

    2.

    3.

- List three reasons a personal self-care practice is important *to you*.

    1.

    2.

    3.

do

Activity 1-1: My Current Self-Care Practice Inventory

- We are quite certain that you already engage in self-care practices, whether you label them as such or not. Think back over the past few years. What do you do to care for yourself when you feel stressed, anxious, or overwhelmed? Do you go for a run? Call a friend? Knit? Knock back a few beers? Do some online shopping? Write down all the activities that you turn to when you need to calm yourself.

- Once you have made this list, put a plus sign next to the activities that you think are helpful and that you would like to include in your self-care tool kit. Put a minus sign next to those that you might want to eliminate or modify, such as self-medicating with food or drink.

Activity 1-2: Self-Care Google Exploration

- This activity is included in the textbook. Google the terms "self-care" and "self-care practices." Expand your search if you're feeling especially ambitious or curious.

- Make a list of some of what pops up. You will find memes, posters, infographics, quotes, research articles, and more. Make a list, or a Pinterest board, of things that intrigue you or resonate with your personality and current self-care practices.

- Which concepts make you think, "*I could get into this*" or "*This makes sense to me*"? What ideas intrigue you or make you want to learn more? These concepts might be your own personal entrées into the study and practice of self-care.

- As you are browsing the internet for self-care practices and ideas, try to categorize each practice into one of the following self-care and wellness categories: physical, mental, emotional, spiritual, intellectual, social, financial, and environmental. Some may fit into more than one category.

Activity 1-3: Try the Big Four

We end Chapter 1 with four of the fundamental self-care practices: checking in with yourself and unclenching when you find tension in your body; staying hydrated; taking deep, restorative breaths; and staying present. Begin to integrate these practices into your daily routine. Use whatever reminder system works best for you, whether it's alarms on your phone, post-it notes, or something else.

reflect & journal

- As you explore self-care practices in your Google search, try to imagine yourself engaging in some of these practices. Are you an athlete or an artist? Do you recoup your energy by being in nature? Is your highest priority staying connected with family and friends?

- What self-care practices would you like to learn more about and consider including in your self-care tool kit?

- Which of the Big Four practices (unclenching, hydration, breathing, being present) come most naturally to you? Which ones will take a little more work? Why?

- As you begin this journey, we want to caution you about comparing yourself to others. Comparing ourselves to others can often feel like a competition and can induce more stress and self-doubt. As you journal about your experiences with self-care, consider a different type of comparison. Compare yourself not to others, but to *you*. Observe the progress you have made. Celebrate your curiosity and willingness to try new things. Stick to it. Ask for help when you need it. Support and acknowledge the progress of others.

2
The Fundamentals of Resilience, Growth, and Wisdom

what

- Read Chapter 2.
- What do we mean by the term “resilience”?
- List three ways that your workplace can foster individual resilience.
    1.
    2.
    3.
- What are the four components of grit, another kind of resilience?
    1.
    2.
    3.
    4.

why

- Why is neuroplasticity important in our ability to become resilient?

- In this chapter, we present two nursing students, Nevin and Pat. Explain in your own words how these two students have learned to approach challenges. Which student do you most closely resemble? Why?

do

Activity 2-1: Foster Positive Emotions

One foundation of well-being is fostering positive emotions. Just as a steady diet of negativity will breed negativity, engaging in activities that make us feel good will help us feel good. Happiness and well-being researcher Barbara Frederickson (Cohn et al., 2009) identified 10 universal positive emotions that we ask you to explore here. For this activity, write down at least one activity or experience that gives rise to each emotion in you. For example, you might feel awe when you see a hawk fly overhead. Perhaps you feel inspiration when you observe an experienced nurse perform a difficult procedure. After identifying what creates positive emotions, the next step is to be intentional about experiencing them. If calling your best friend generates feelings of love, call your best friend more often. If a particular song makes you feel joyful, listen to that song!

Emotion	Activity
Joy	
Gratitude	
Serenity	
Interest	
Hope	
Pride	
Amusement	
Inspiration	
Awe	
Love	

Activity 2-2: Savor the Moment

Rick Hanson (2018) argues that we must "sit with" positive emotions to rewire our brains for resilience. In Chapter 2, we provided a hypothetical list of daily opportunities to savor positive emotions. For at least one day, be very intentional about savoring positive moments, from the moment you wake up until you fall asleep at night. Write down as many of these moments as possible. After this one-day exercise, remind yourself to continue savoring positive emotions.

reflect & journal

- How will you be able to maintain this practice of fostering positive emotions and savoring them once you are in clinical practice? What techniques and strategies can you use to help build these activities into your daily and weekly routine?

- We all know someone, either personally or from the news or history books, who has overcome extreme adversity and grown wiser as a result of their experience. In the textbook, we include Congressman John Lewis, Malala Yousafzai, and the Marjorie Stoneman Douglas High School students as examples of individuals who were able to transform their pain into wisdom. Who do you consider wise? Why do you consider them to be wise? What qualities do they exhibit? Did they overcome adversity as part of their journey to wisdom?

- How does it feel to be intentional about fostering and savoring positive emotions? Is this a new experience for you? Is it something that you can continue to do? Why or why not?

- You are capable. You are strong. You are wise. You will become more able, strong, and wise as you learn and grow. Say it aloud to yourself: "I am capable. I am strong. I am wise." Believe it.

references

Cohn, M. A., Fredrickson, B. L., Brown, S. L., Mikels, J. A., & Conway, A. M. (2009). Happiness unpacked: Positive emotions increase life satisfaction by building resilience. *Emotion*, 9(3), 361–368. https://doi.org/10.1037/a0015952

Hanson, R. (2018). *Resilient: How to grow an unshakable core of calm, strength, and happiness.* Harmony Books.

3

Developing a Resilient Mindset Using Appreciative Practices

what

- Read Chapter 3.
- What is the negativity bias? Give some examples of this bias in your own life.
- What are some of the well-being benefits of positive activities?
- Explain two of the theoretical principles (constructionist, poetic, positive, simultaneity, anticipatory) of Appreciative Inquiry in your own words.

why

In this chapter, the authors discuss the importance of "choosing our focus." Explain what this entails and why it matters. (You may want to refer back to the Nevin and Pat examples in Chapter 2.)

do

Activity 3-1: Choose Language With Care

As the authors explain, language creates our reality. Observe the choices that people make with language. How does naming something a certain way change words' impact? Pay attention to your own language choices. Did you learn to use certain words in your childhood that seem problematic today?

Activity 3-2: Reframing

What we choose to focus on becomes our fate (Whitney & Trosten-Bloom, 2003). Reframing is the capacity to intentionally explore new ways of seeing to experience the best of what is. Think of something that is annoying, sad, disappointing, or challenging. Now reframe this situation to find the best of what is. For example, you may have a long walk to your campus or hospital. You could reframe this by realizing that the walk is an opportunity for exercise, time to listen to music, or a chance to prepare for or decompress from your day.

Activity 3-3: Gratitude Practice

A growing body of research finds that a simple gratitude practice can improve well-being among nurses and other healthcare workers (Sexton & Adair, 2019). Commit to taking time at the end of each day to write down three good things that happened to you during the day. These can be exciting events such as acing an exam or receiving a job offer, but most likely, they will be more humble moments. You might appreciate a delicious meal, an unexpected connection with a friend, a nap, or a sunny day.

You may choose to write your three good things in a small notebook, on your phone, or on your laptop. The most important thing is to do it regularly for at least 10 days. You will begin to notice that throughout the day, your attention and thoughts will be drawn toward those good things around you and away from those things that produce negative feelings.

If you would like to take this exercise a step further, pick one good thing each day and reflect on the people and events that made that good thing possible. For example, if you are grateful for a hot cup of coffee, think about the barista who made it to work that day and the workers who manufactured the cups; you will increase your sense of connection with the world around you.

Activity 3-4: Positivity Portfolio

A positivity portfolio is a collection of objects, words, or photos that stirs positive emotions in the viewer or reader. Positivity portfolios are more common than we realize. A collection of photos, plants, and seashells on someone's desk is a positivity portfolio. A group of refrigerator magnets that reminds a family of their travels together is a positivity portfolio. A collection of favorite quotes and a laptop or water bottle covered in stickers are positivity portfolios. A playlist can be a positivity portfolio. Create your own portfolio in any way you choose. All that matters is that you create a collection of items that makes you feel a positive emotion, such as happiness, contentment, or peace.

Activity 3-5: Vision Board

We move toward the image of the future that we hold in our heads, and the more positive that vision, the more positive our future. Remember the story of Ryan Speedo Green, the young man who saw his first opera at the Met and visualized himself performing on that same stage someday. Creating positive visions of our future is a remarkably powerful tool.

To create a vision board, gather a stack of old magazines, scissors, a piece of cardstock or cardboard, and a glue stick. Give yourself at least an hour (set a timer) to flip through the magazines and cut out photos and words that represent the future you are seeking. Relax. What dreams do you have for yourself? (This exercise can be done for the upcoming year or a longer time frame, whichever seems best to you.) Cut and glue the pictures to your cardstock, and keep the collage somewhere where you can see it regularly.

Activity 3-6: Vision Board, With No Glue

Are you trying to make a difficult decision about your future? Is there something you desire, but you are having trouble achieving it? Create a quiet space and give yourself at least a half hour to do this activity. Visualize your life one year from now. What does it look like? The power is in the details. Imagine yourself waking up in the morning. Where are you? What do you eat for breakfast? Is someone with you, or are you alone? Go through your entire day in this future life, focusing on your work, your friends, the activities of your day. *Remember—details, details, details.* Pay attention to how you feel. On a piece of paper, write down as many details as you can remember.

reflect & journal

- We hope this chapter gave you a lot of ideas and food for thought. Which activities were the most helpful? Were any so compelling that you think you would be able to include them in your self-care tool kit?

- "Our focus is our fate." Spend a few moments writing about your own focus and how it affects your well-being in the short and long term.

references

Sexton, J. B., & Adair, K. C. (2019). Forty-five good things: A prospective pilot study of the Three Good Things well-being intervention in the USA for healthcare worker emotional exhaustion, depression, work-life balance and happiness. *BMJ Open, 9*(3), e022695. https://doi.org/10.1136/bmjopen-2018-022695

Whitney, D., & Trosten-Bloom, A. (2003). *The power of Appreciative Inquiry: A practical guide to positive change.* Berrett-Koehler Publishers, Inc.

4

The Community Resiliency Model (CRM)® Approach to Mental Wellness for Nursing Students and New Graduate Nurses

what

- Read Chapter 4.
- Describe the difference between the sympathetic and parasympathetic nervous systems.

- What is the resilient zone? What can cause someone to "bounce out" of their resilient zone? What are the differences between the high zone and the low zone?

- List the six skills that make up the Community Resilience Model (CRM)®.'

1.

2.

3.

4.

5.

6.

why

The textbook includes many approaches to self-care in clinical practice. What differentiates the CRM from other self-care techniques (both those included in this book and traditional self-care activities)? Why is CRM especially appropriate for nurses?

do

Activities to help you develop all six CRM skills are described in detail in Chapter 4 of the textbook.

Activity 4-1: Tracking

Tracking directs our conscious awareness toward positive or neutral sensations in our body (Miller-Karas, 2015). Tracking is the foundation for the other CRM skills and is closely related to many other practices described in the textbook. You can practice tracking by shifting your awareness and paying attention to your five senses. Identifying and sensing these pleasant or neutral sensations decrease the body's tendency to focus so closely on the discomfort messages.

Notice things that you can see, hear, smell, taste, and feel. Notice feelings inside your body, such as tension, thirst, and tingling. Notice your breathing. Is it fast or slow? Deep or shallow?

Activity 4-2: Resourcing

Resourcing uses the first skill, tracking, to help you build a sense of internal strength. A powerful tool, resourcing is like a strong muscle that reinforces your own sense of capability and purpose. Your *internal resources* can be many things: your values or beliefs; a wonderful quality, talent, or ability; or a significant experience or moment in your life. Your *external resources* may include happy memories, people, places, or things that bring you support, calm, or peace (Miller-Karas, 2015). They could be hobbies, social groups, and animals. *Imagined resources* are those that are brought to mind from experiences yet to be, like a daydream or a wished-for image or thought.

Resourcing is akin to establishing a new pathway in the limbic system or etching a positive template in the mind. We are essentially using our own nervous system to calm our nervous system. A resource is like a template you can access anytime, and like a muscle, its strength grows with repeated use. You can draw on your resource any time, and under times of stress, you can use your resource to counter any existing negative templates that are the natural stress default in your brain (Vaish et al., 2008). When you experience future stress, you can purposefully access your resource and return to the resilient zone as your central nervous system begins to reset and release tension.

Take a moment to identify a resource that you'd like to try out. It could be a memory, idea, place, or person associated with calm, comfort, and safety. Maybe it is walking along a beach or jogging through a park. If you're a musician, maybe your resource is mentally rehearsing a song or remembering a time you played music with friends. For artists, a resource might be visualizing the next painting or sculpture they will create or walking through a museum. Everyone's resource is different, but it should evoke calm and pleasant feelings.

Now that you have decided on a resource to try, take a moment to describe three or four aspects of the resource in your mind. Write down what comes to mind. As with the visualization exercise in the previous chapter, it is important to be as descriptive and detailed as possible. Your goal is to paint a rich picture that touches all your senses. This elaboration is called *resource intensification*, a way to deepen the resource with sensory details that help the resource become more potent. As you think about your resource, what do you notice happening on the inside of your body (*heart rate, breathing, changes in muscles, fullness, warmth, lightness*)? Do you notice any movement on the outside of your body (*smiles, gestures, posture changes*)? Notice if the sensations are pleasant, unpleasant, or neutral.

Once you have found these pleasant or neutral sensations, stay with them for about 12–20 seconds. There is no rush to get back to daily life. Rather, take your time to firmly establish this resource. Staying with it for a period will strengthen your newfound resilience pathway. Revisit your resource periodically to get used to relying on it. Resourcing is a muscle you can stretch and strengthen anytime you want to stay in your resilient zone or get back inside your best self.

Activity 4-3: Grounding, Gesturing, Help Now!, and Shift and Stay

Please refer to the textbook for detailed instructions on learning these additional four CRM skills.

reflect & journal

- Think about what you are like when you are in your personal resilient zone. Describe your "best-self" in that zone. What do you feel like? What keeps you in that zone, and what in your life can pull you out of it?

- Hopefully you have begun to master the six CRM skills. What do you think they can contribute to your current and future well-being?

- The authors begin their chapter with a quote by Elaine Miller-Karas, the creator of the CRM: "When we bring awareness to the inner wisdom of our bodies, wellbeing can grow, even in times of great suffering. Moments of gratitude can be seen and sensed." Take a few moments to reflect on the connection between "awareness to the wisdom of our bodies" and well-being.

references

Miller-Karas, E. (2015). *Building resilience to trauma: The trauma and community resiliency models.* Routledge.

Vaish, A., Grossmann, T., & Woodward, A. (2008). Not all emotions are created equal: The negativity bias in social-emotional development. *Psychological Bulletin*, *134*(3), 383–403. https://doi.org/10.1037/0033-2909.134.3.383

section II

The Mind of a Nurse

5

Self-Care, Community Care, and Resilience Among Underrepresented Minority Nursing Professionals and Students

what

- Read Chapter 5.
- Describe at least five unique challenges underrepresented minority (URM) nurses face.

    1.

    2.

    3.

    4.

    5.

- The author states that "Nurses' experiences of emotional labor are not only gendered but also racialized." Explain what she means by this.

- What unique barriers to self-care do URM nurses face?

- What unique strengths might URM nurses bring to their professional experience?

why

Why is communal care a potentially more effective strategy for well-being than self-care?

do

Activity 5-1: Responding to Discriminatory Behavior: Individuals

Have you experienced or observed the racial or ethnic identity-based discriminative experiences during your training? If so, what was your response or the response of others? If possible, gather in a group of four to five peers, establish expectations for students to safely share their experiences, and begin this conversation. Give yourselves time to make sure that all voices are heard.

Activity 5-2: Responding to Discriminatory Behavior: Healthcare Institutions

Reflect on and discuss with your peers how healthcare institutions can address the issues URM nursing professionals and students experience. What types of resources are available in your institution that might help address these issues? Are there any structural and policy changes you would like to see?

Generate a list of policy and health system changes your team envisions that would build equity, inclusion, and diversity into your school or workplace.

reflect & journal

- Think about examples of communal care in your own life and how they have had an impact on your well-being. Now consider ways that communal care and similar well-being benefits can be cultivated in healthcare organizations. What would our healthcare organizations look like, and in what ways would they focus on diversity, inclusion, and equity?

- Dr. Çayir selected this quote by Maya Angelou to open her chapter: "My mission in life is not merely to survive, but to thrive; and to do so with some passion, some compassion, some humor, and some style." Imagine yourself in your role as a nurse. In what ways will you embody these qualities—passion, compassion, humor, and style—into your work and life?

6
Self-Care for LGBTQIA+ Nursing Students

what

- Read Chapter 6.
- List the additional stressors faced by LGBTQIA+ nursing students.

- Given these additional stressors, self-care strategies are vitally important for the LGBTQIA+ nursing student. Describe the four LGBTQIA+-specific self-care strategies that the author suggests in this chapter.

    1.

    2.

    3.

    4.

why

This chapter opens with the famous quote by Audre Lorde: "Caring for myself is not self-indulgence, it is self-preservation, and that is an act of political warfare" (Lorde, 1988, p. 205). Why is caring for oneself an act of political warfare?

do

Activity 6-1: The Importance of Being Seen

If you identify as LGBTQIA+, how did it feel reading a chapter that was written in a voice that was clearly speaking to you? Think of times in your life when you have felt seen. What specific behaviors on the part of others make you feel this way?

If you identify as heterosexual and cisgender, how did it feel reading a chapter that was written in a voice that was clearly speaking to someone other than you? In what ways did the author express her compassion and understanding for her readers? Think of times in your life when you have felt seen for who you truly are. What specific behaviors on the part of others make you feel this way?

reflect & journal

- In what ways can you be more intentional about helping others feel truly seen by you?

- Identity is complex—LGBTQIA+ nursing students aren't *just* LGBTQIA+. They hold other identities simultaneously: Black, Latinx, Indigenous/Native, Jewish, Christian, Muslim, athiest, first generation college student, and so on. LGBTQIA+ nursing students may also be persons with ability status that informs how they identify themselves, or persons for whom English is the second language they learned.

- What identities do you hold? How do you care for each of those identities?

reference

Lorde, A. (1988). *A burst of light: And other essays.* Courier Dover Publications.

7

Nursing Our Identities: Self-Compassion and Intersectionality

what

- Read Chapter 7.
- Explain the differences between self-worth, self-esteem, and self-compassion as described in this chapter.

- What are the three components of self-compassion?

    1.

    2.

    3.

- What are the specific benefits of self-compassion?

why

This chapter deepens our examination of the diversity of self-care practices. Why is our culture or family heritage so important to our personal well-being?

do

Activity 7-1: Cultural Heritage and Self-Care

As a form of self-care and self-compassion, the author discovered, "To know ourselves requires an understanding of all the forces that have shaped us—notably, the distant past." Based on your own and your family's cultural traditions and experiences, what self-care do you practice that might not be included in the traditional self-care literature?

Are there self-care practices described in the traditional self-care literature or this book that may not be culturally appropriate for you?

Activity 7-2: Shaping Our Self-Worth

Our sense of self-worth is a combination of self-esteem and self-compassion and is paramount in the discussion of self-care throughout the chapter. Take time to identify and list the myriad factors that shape your sense of self-worth. What factors are external (for example, approval of others), and which are internal?

reflect & journal

- When the author turned to historical research as a form of self-care, this illustrates an excellent example of "resourcing," as described in Chapter 4. What forms of resourcing do you rely on now? What additional forms could you add to your tool kit?

- The chapter author exposed vulnerability by sharing experiences of what he considered "failures." Write about a time when you have failed. How did you move through that adversity? How did you care for yourself or show yourself compassion? What would you say to that earlier version of yourself now?

8
Narrative Practices

what

- Read Chapter 8.
- This chapter is about paying attention. How can narrative practices, and other activities that foster deep awareness, help you become a better clinician?

- Describe the three levels of resonance, or caring: sympathetic, empathetic, and compassionate.

why

In considering our ability to reflect, defract, and deflect emotions, why is awareness of this phenomenon so important to nurses? What examples can you provide?

do

Activity 8-1: Visual Arts

In groups of three or four, collectively select a famous painting or sculpture. You may consider browsing websites of a local art museum to find images on the web. Once you find the image, designate one person in the group to prompt discussion questions about the image. (This exercise may certainly be done on your own, but it is an excellent group activity.) Here is a list of museum websites:

- **The Tate Modern:** https://www.tate.org.uk
- **The Metropolitan Museum of Art:** https://www.metmuseum.org
- **Museo Botero:** https://www.banrepcultural.org/bogota/museo-botero
- **The National Bardo Museum:** http://www.bardomuseum.tn

- **Tokyo National Museum:** https://www.tnm.jp/?lang=en
- **National Museum Australia:** https://www.nma.gov.au

Ask the following questions of the group, and allow time for everyone to respond.

1. What comes to mind first when you see this image?

2. What is the first feeling (if any) that comes up for you?

3. Look closely now at the textures of the image. What do you see?

4. Look closely now at the colors in the image. What do you see?

5. What do you think the artist was trying to say with this piece of work?

6. If you could meet the artist right now, what would you tell them about this work?

Activity 8-2: Capturing Your Own Experience in Art

Think of a patient encounter or healthcare experience that had meaning to you. Select an art form—prose or poetry writing, painting, drawing, collage, music, photography—and convey your experience of this encounter. Relax and enjoy this process. There is no right or wrong, good or bad.

reflect & journal

- In this chapter, the author writes, "That calling [to become a nurse] is at the core of our lived experience. Uniquely ours, lived experience is an important aspect of our lives to examine because, from it, we will know ourselves better. In knowing ourselves better, we'll better understand our own, individual and critical self-care needs." Write about your calling to become a nurse. What is your story?

- Select a narrative of health, illness, or healing to read. You may choose one included in this chapter (for example, *Violation*, *When Breath Becomes Air*, *Fun Home),* or choose one of the many others that have been written. If an entire book feels daunting, select an essay or short story. Use the narrative practice skills we have discussed to reflect on the work you chose. How did the work make you feel? How did it change you? What did it convey about the author and their experience of health, illness, or healing?

9

Mindful Compassion: A Life in Practice

what

- Read Chapter 9.
- Describe *beginner's mind.* How do we foster it? What are the barriers to it? How can this fresh perspective make us more compassionate in our work?

why

The author uses mindfulness and the practices described in the chapter to make him a more compassionate physician. Why is this ability important to his well-being?

do

Activity 9-1: Developing Beginner's Mind

At the heart of beginner's mind is the ability to see things with fresh eyes, even (or especially) things that we take for granted, that blend into the background of our everyday lives. For at least one day, be intentional about noticing the everyday objects, buildings, natural elements, and people of your life with fresh eyes. What changes? In Chapter 3, we talked about an "appreciative eye," that there is beauty in everything. Do you notice more beauty when you use a beginner's mind?

Activity 9-2: Developing Compassion

Now that you have gotten a taste of beginner's mind, try taking this technique a step further. View one of the paintings the author suggests in his chapter: Van Gogh's *Sorrowing Old Man* (*At Eternity's Gate*), Leo Twiggs's *Hooded*, Goya's *Self Portrait with Dr. Arrieta*, and Sir Luke Fildes's *The Doctor*.

Take a few moments to look at the painting, allowing yourself to empathically resonate and allowing compassion to arise. Notice what you observe in the painting. Notice what you observe in yourself. Notice what you would say or do if you met the people as they are depicted in these photographs.

Activity 9-3: Waiting Room Observation

Set aside an hour to sit in a busy waiting area. This can be in a hospital, but it can also be a department of motor vehicles, train station, or airport. Spend this time focusing your attention on one individual at a time. Try to imagine what their day has been like so far. Where did they sleep? What did they consume for breakfast? Why are they in this particular space, and how did they get here? What are they worried about? What might they be looking forward to? Whom do they love? Who loves them? Your conclusions do not have to be factual or "correct"; they simply need to be details that humanize the individuals you observe.

reflect & journal

- The chapter author includes this Blaise Pascal quote: "In difficult times carry something beautiful in your heart" (Goodreads, n.d.). What does Pascal mean by this? Why did the author include it?

- Do you believe it is possible to feel compassion toward someone whom you dislike or even despise? Why or why not?

- Write, write, write, write. When you have a meaningful encounter, positive or negative, take the time to process it through writing. It doesn't have to be perfect, but let the words flow. Then let it go. See what you learn.

reference

Goodreads. (n.d.). *Blaise Pascal quotes.* https://www.goodreads.com/quotes/410084-in-difficult-times-carry-something-beautiful-in-your-heart

10
Self-Care and Systemic Change: What You Need to Know

what

- Read Chapter 10.
- There are pitfalls to focusing on individual self-care above all else. What are the author's concerns about this?
- Explain moral distress in your own words. Provide at least one example.
- What is the #selfcare movement? Why is it potentially harmful for true well-being?

why

- Why is the "mythology of heroic, self-sacrificing women who cared for the sick" problematic for the well-being of today's nurses?

do

Activity 10-1: The Mythology of Nursing

This chapter links the origin myths and stereotypes of nursing to many of the underlying systemic issues in healthcare today. Dig a little deeper into this notion of potentially harmful perceptions of nursing and nurses. What misperceptions have you personally encountered? What stereotypes did you grow up with? Have these stereotypical images changed since you've become a nursing student?

Activity 10-2: #selfcare

In Chapter 1, we invited you to do a Google search of self-care practices. Our goal was to give you a broad sense of the self-care activities and options available to you as you begin this journey. We suggested that you view your search results through a personal lens: What practices were appealing to you? Which were you curious to learn more about? Now we invite you to revisit your Google search, or do another one, and look at the search results through the #selfcare lens. Which create unrealistic expectations? Which may not be based in good science? Which promote unhelpful stereotypes? Which are actually ridiculous? Which might be harmful?

reflect & journal

- Imagine yourself in an unhealthy work environment. (We hope this doesn't happen to you.) What would you do in that situation? What options might you have?

- It is discouraging to think that your workplace may not prioritize the well-being of its employees. As we wrote in the editors' introduction to the textbook chapter, there is a tension between self-care and institutional responsibility. Give yourself some time and space to reflect and write on this difficult issue.

11

Strengths-Based Self-Care: Good Enough, Strong Enough, Wise Enough

what

- Read Chapter 11.
- What is the "victim narrative"? How can it be detrimental to well-being?
- Explain posttraumatic growth (PTG) in your own words.
- What are the five elements of PTG?

    1.

    2.

    3.

    4.

    5.

- List the five aspects of high emotional intelligence.

    1.

    2.

    3.

    4.

    5.

why

Why might "not taking it personally" be one of the most valuable tools in your self-care tool kit?

do

Activity 11-1: Growth From Trauma

Take some time to read about a person you admire. They could be a civil rights or political leader, community advocate, artist, scientist, businessperson, or celebrity. You might choose a nurse, friend, or loved one. As you learn about this person, consider any trauma that they experienced. How did that trauma lead to transformation and growth? What strengths did they draw on to help them navigate the traumatic event?

Activity 11-2: Inherent Strengths Inventory

This chapter contends that we all have inherent strengths, and we can build on these strengths as a form of self-care. In other words, we don't have to begin from scratch, and we don't have to learn everything anew. We each have qualities and characteristics that will help us navigate adversity, grow, and maintain our well-being. We invite you to create your own strengths inventory. Consider traits that are included in this chapter, but we encourage you to expand your view to include other qualities as well.

reflect & journal

How have you moved through adversity or trauma in your life? How did that experience transform you, in good ways and bad?

section III
The Body and Spirit of a Nurse

12
Reclaiming, Recalling, and Remembering: Spirituality and Self-Care

what

- Read Chapter 12.
- How does this author define "spirituality"?

- What does the author mean by "vocation"?

- Describe the term "paradoxical thinking," and give three examples.

why

Why is it important to acknowledge and talk about "our true selves"?

do

Activity 12-1: Defining a Belief System

Consider your own belief system or your guiding principles, and write answers to the following questions.

- Who, or what, encouraged you to believe as you do? What in your own life narrative has led you to these beliefs?

- Are your beliefs based on a traditional spiritual practice or something else?

- What specifically are your guiding principles?

- How do your guiding principles affect your daily living? (This could include decision-making, self-care, or simply the way you show up in the world.)

- How do you nurture your spiritual practice or belief system?

- Tell a story about a time that your spiritual practice allowed you to move through a challenging time to a place of peace, compassion, love, or hope.

reflect & journal

- How will your values or beliefs guide your professional role as a nurse?

- The author includes a quote by Parker Palmer (2000) who says we will find our vocation by accepting the "treasure of true self" we already possess. He encourages us to listen for and nurture that true self. Do you think you know who your true self is?

reference

Palmer, P. (2000). *Let your life speak.* Jossey-Bass.

13
Sleep, Exercise, and Nutrition: Self-Care the Kaizen Way

what

- Read Chapter 13.
- Explain the philosophy of Kaizen. How does it relate to a self-care practice?
- List six nonpharmacological sleep aids.

    1.

    2.

    3.

    4.

    5.

    6.

- What are some of the well-being benefits of exercise?
- What are some of the well-being benefits of sexual activity?
- What are the barriers to healthy, nutritious eating faced by many nurses? (You may want to refer to Chapter 1 in the textbook as well.)

why

There are so many voices (experts and otherwise) telling us what to eat to maintain good health. In determining your own nutrition choices, who is the most important expert and why?

do

Activity 13-1: The Sleep-Exercise-Nutrition Triangle

This is an exercise to foster awareness of the connection between the three sides of the sleep-exercise-nutrition triangle and to help you pay attention to your own physical well-being. For seven days, keep track of your sleep, physical activity, and nutrition with simple +, -, or = signs: + indicates that you feel you did well in caring for yourself and meeting your physical needs; – indicates that you think you could have done better; and = indicates you aren't sure, or you are simply satisfied but not impressed. If you'd prefer, you may provide more detailed information in your chart, but our goal is to keep things simple.

Day	Sleep	Exercise	Nutrition	Notes
Example	+	-	=	**Pouring rain; couldn't run** **Ate ok; didn't snack**
1				
2				
3				
4				
5				
6				
7				

After seven days, can you see any patterns? If you had poor sleep on certain days, did exercise and nutrition suffer on those days, too? Are you consistently getting enough sleep but not enough exercise? Describe all the patterns that you notice. What factors had an impact on your physical self-care during this week?

Activity 13-2: Paying Attention

As you went through the week charting your physical self-care, we expect that you may have been paying close attention to your body in a new way. What kinds of things did you notice? What messages did your body send you? For example, how did your body feel after drinking beverages that contain sugar, caffeine, or alcohol?

Activity 13-3: The Kaizen Way

Consider what you learned this week using a Kaizen mindset. Where do you see opportunities for small steps that might result in change? Think about the sleep-exercise-nutrition triad, and identify one small change you can make. Commit to it for 10 days. We offer a few suggestions to get you thinking. Of course, refer to the *Self-Care* textbook and other sources for ideas.

- Take the stairs instead of using the elevator.
- Turn off all screens 15 minutes before you lie down to sleep.
- Eat vegetarian for one meal a day.
- Pack healthy snacks—fruit, sugar-free yogurt, trail mix—in your backpack.
- Park farther away and walk.
- Use a sleep app to help you fall asleep.
- Eat one meal each day slowly and mindfully.
- Drink a glass of water first thing in the morning.

If this exercise resonates with you, consider adding one small change to the mix each week. Notice what larger changes begin to happen in your life.

reflect & journal

- What if, in this moment, you are good enough? We can say with surety that you *are* good enough. This chapter is not about being good or bad, but about caring for yourself, especially your physical self. This chapter is about paying attention to your body so that you can respond to its needs. If your body needs something (more sleep, more movement, better fuel), you can make those changes slowly, one at a time.

- Write down all the reasons that you want to care for your body.

14

Six Steps to Compassion: Practicing T'ai Chi in a Healthcare Setting

what

- Read Chapter 14.
- T'ai Chi is considered an internal martial art. How does T'ai Chi differ from other fitness programs?

- List at least six of the health benefits of T'ai Chi.

1.

2.

3.

4.

5.

6.

why

Why might a health system consider offering T'ai Chi classes for its staff? What benefits might result?

do

Activity 14-1: Try T'ai Chi

We encourage you to avail yourself of a T'ai Chi class. Explore a T'ai Chi center in your local area, if possible. Some of author Master Hiromi Hangai Johnson's teachings can be found at: https://www.charlottesvilletaichi.org/classes/student-resources/. You can also take online classes; some are free.

Activity 14-2: Sensing the Gap

This chapter describes something that we often refer to as the space between stimulus and response. Something happens to you—someone bumps into you, a friend annoys you, or a patient complains—and you have a brief moment when you may choose how to respond. That gap—that moment when we have a choice—provides more power and control than many of us realize. We have the freedom to choose our response to everything and everyone we encounter.

The chapter authors write that, "Rather than trying to smooth over gaps by eliminating them, T'ai Chi helps people notice the gaps and draws attention to their productive possibilities."

For today, notice the gaps. Notice your power to choose.

reflect & journal

- The authors write, "There is always some sort of sensation in your body, but you're just not noticing it. If you are being observant about yourself, that will affect other people." This is yet another reminder to pay attention, in this case to your body. What sensations are you feeling now? Check in with yourself as often as you can today.

15
Reflections on Self-Care and Your Clinical Practice

what

- Read Chapter 15.
- How does this author create in-the-moment self-care opportunities in the middle of a busy clinical practice?
- What is a transition ritual?
- What does the author mean when she writes about "set an intention" or "intention setting"?

why

Why does the author sometimes cringe when she looks back on her early days as a nurse?

do

Activity 15-1: Transition Rituals

The chapter author uses journaling as a transition activity before and after her shifts. We know other nurses who use prayer, exercise, music, or meditation to help them prepare or decompress. What transition rituals have you used in the past, even if you didn't name them as such? Try at least one transition ritual this week as you come and go to school or your clinical rotations.

Activity 15-2: To-Be-Joyful (*not* a To-Do) List

In a chapter sidebar, Jennifer shares ways that she cares for herself on her days off. One way is to make a list of activities; the list makes her feel productive and allows her to intentionally focus on self-care. "This list keeps me reminded of activities outside of work that help me de-stress and stay organized. As I cross these tasks off my list, I earn my sense of productivity and feel ready to give back to others around me."

Imagine that you have all the time in the world to do things that make you happy. Write a list of these activities.

Activity 15-3: Frames of Reference

Review the author's description of her frames of reference, her guiding principles for showing up as a nurse. What frames of reference do you think would serve you well in your clinical practice? How do they build on the guiding principles that you live by today?

reflect & journal

- The textbook has focused a lot of attention on physical self-awareness—noticing when you are tense, tired, thirsty, and more. This chapter approaches self-awareness from a different perspective. What kind of self-awareness makes the author the kind of nurse that she is?

- We especially love the author's description of Tonglen practice and how she uses the practice to foster loving-kindness toward those she encounters in her practice. We encourage you to learn more about this practice as a way to "set your intentions" toward your patients.

- The chapter author closes by writing about boundaries as a form of self-care. What are your boundaries in your life today? What additional boundaries would you like to establish?

section IV
The Transition to Nursing Practice

16
Supportive Professional Relationships: Mentoring and Nurse Residency Programs

what

- Read Chapter 16.
- List the seven major challenges that newly licensed registered nurses face.

    1.

    2.

    3.

    4.

    5.

    6.

    7.

- What are the goals of transition to practice nurse residency programs?

- Describe the benefits of having a mentor.

- A nurse mentor can serve as a coach, counselor, confidant, encourager, friend, visionary, and resource. What roles should a mentor *not* embrace?

why

Why should nurses and mentors set specific goals, and what might they entail?

do

Activity 16-1: Investigate NRPs

Spend some time researching hospitals or health systems and their nurse residency programs (NRPs). Do they meet all of the criteria outlined in this chapter, such as being 9 to 12 months long, having an evidence-based curriculum, and so on? Are they accredited by the Commission on Collegiate Nursing Education (CCNE) or the American Nurses Credentialing Center (ANCC)? Do they offer evidence-based practice projects? (Review the NRP checklist at the end of the chapter.)

Activity 16-2: S.M.A.R.T. Goal Setting

Goal setting is an important part of the mentoring experience for both the mentee and the mentor. But what is a good goal? What are some criteria by which you can assess the strength of a goal? One way to structure goals is by using the S.M.A.R.T. goal approach. S.M.A.R.T. stands for Specific, Measurable, Attainable, Relevant, and Time-based. Consider one goal for yourself that you can achieve this month. It can be anything related to school, work, home, or self-care. In the following table, complete a S.M.A.R.T. diagram for your goal. Enter the name of your goal and generate the S.M.A.R.T. steps you will take to achieve it. Once you write this goal down, take steps toward completing it.

Name of Goal:	Responses:
Specific: Write details about what this goal entails.	
Measurable: Write exactly how you will measure accomplishment of this goal.	
Achievable: Is this goal achievable? How do you know? What have you achieved before this point that will help you know you can reach this one?	
Relevant: Write how this goal aligns with who you are, your personal beliefs, and your larger goals in life.	
Time-based: What is the realistic time frame during which you can begin to work on this goal and when you plan to achieve it? Are there milestones or checkpoints along the way that you can list to hit while you are achieving this goal?	

reflect & journal

- It's not all about the mentor. It is also the mentee's responsibility to collaborate effectively with the mentor and develop a trusting relationship. Zachary (2012) came up with nine essential mentee skills, listed next. Consider your own skills for each of these areas. Where are your strengths, and where might you need some improvement? What might you do to strengthen some of these skills?

    1. Ability to receive and give feedback

    2. Self-directed

    3. Open communicator

    4. Taking initiative

    5. Valuing self-reflection

    6. Ability to listen

    7. Ability to follow through

    8. Relationship building

    9. Ability to set goals

- In today's fast-paced "gig economy," some say that mentoring in nursing may be a dying art. How can you serve as a mentor to others today and in the future? Perhaps you are already serving in a mentoring role, either formal or informal. How can you reignite the art of mentoring?

reference

Zachary, L. J. (2012). *The mentor's guide* (2nd ed.). John Wiley & Sons, Inc. Jossey-Bass. San Francisco.

17
Healthy Work Environment: How to Choose One for Your First Job

what

- Read Chapter 17.
- List the six standards for establishing and sustaining a healthy work environment (HWE).

  1.

  2.

  3.

  4.

  5.

  6.

- "Skilled communication" is a broad standard that includes a range of important topics. List at least five aspects of skilled communication in a healthy work environment.
- What distinguishes the Daisy Award as a meaningful form of recognition for nurses?

why

Why are some environments healthier than others? What factors have you observed in clinical settings that have led you to say, "This would be a good place to work," or "This is not a place I would like to work"?

do

Activity 17-1: Identifying Priorities for Your First Job

Reflect on the priorities you might consider when choosing your first job in nursing. Rank the six following criteria on level of importance from 1 to 7, where 1 has the highest importance to you and 7 has the lowest, at least in the early stages of your career. Use the table to rank these items, and briefly describe your reasoning or considerations for each ranking. We have included additional rows for you to add other priorities, if needed.

Priority	Rank (1–7)	Reasons for Ranking/Factors to Consider
Geographic location		
Specialty		
Reputation of organization		
Proximity to family and friends		
Availability or quality of a nurse residency program		
Type of hospital: teaching vs. community or private		
"Feel"/support of the work environment		
Other priority		
Other priority		

Activity 17-2: Rocking the Interview

One strategy to land that first exciting position in your top hospital and unit is to shine in the interview. Below are several questions to consider. As you read through the list, consider what to add, and perhaps put a star next to the ones that underscore your most important values and priorities. We have used the HWE Standards to frame these as well as Jennifer Hargreaves's and Christine Pabico's 2020 article, "How to Choose Your First Nursing Job Wisely." They acknowledge that nurse leaders will carefully interview you to make sure you are the right fit. You should be doing the same interviewing: Is this hospital the right fit for you? Their suggestions come from the American Nurses Credentialing Center Pathway to Excellence Interview Tool (Hargreaves & Pabico, 2020).

Interview Questions to Ask

1. Does your organization use the AACN Standards for an HWE? (Bring a copy to the interview.)
2. Is there Magnet® designation? Beacon units?
3. How long is the nurse residency program? What are the components?

4. Describe the orientation program. Is there a potential to increase it if needed?
5. What are the nurse turnover/retention and nurse vacancy rates for the past two years?
6. What do nurses state as their reason for leaving?
7. Are there programs for nursing staff development such as Crucial Conversations, patient safety, and clinical topics? Are these programs interprofessional, including physicians and other disciplines?
8. Describe the shared governance program and the committees where staff nurses are engaged.
9. What happens when there is conflict or disrespect? Are there policies in place based upon the ANA recommendations?
10. How visible is the nurse manager on the unit? Do they wear scrubs, at least some of the time?
11. What are the biggest challenges nurses face each day? How is the nurse staffing determined? Has there been turnover in the nursing leadership recently?
12. Describe the clinical ladder. Are there awards for nurses? Is the hospital signed on to provide the Daisy Award to nurses?
13. What are the hospital's most notable successes?
14. Describe the programs for nurse well-being.

reflect & journal

- Choosing your first nursing job probably feels stressful, but we hope this chapter has helped you feel a little less so. What are your concerns, fears, and worries about your first job? What elements of your first work environment might alleviate some of those concerns?
- This might be a good time to encourage you to reflect on all the accomplishments you have already achieved, all the challenges you have met with grace and energy, and the many skills you have mastered. Set a timer for 10 minutes, and make a list of all you are proud of about yourself. Write quickly, and do not think too much. Just write.
- The importance of "meaningful recognition" came to the fore during the COVID-19 pandemic. Citizens applauded healthcare workers during shift changes. We left our Christmas lights up through the winter to acknowledge their service. Many were celebrated as "heroes." Yet in many hospitals, nurses felt the sting of "*unmeaningful* recognition," such as free pizzas, buttons, or t-shirts. We often heard nurses say something like, "Don't tell me I'm a hero. Just wear your damn mask." What really *is* meaningful recognition? Does it depend on the circumstances? On the individual nurse? What meaningful recognition have you received or would you like to receive?

reference

Hargreaves, J., & Pabico, C. (2020). How to choose your first nursing job wisely. *American Nurse Journal, 15*(5), 30–31.

18

Self-Care for Humanitarian Aid Workers

what

- Read Chapter 18.
- What are the global and humanitarian crises that give rise to the need to deploy healthcare workers?
- What are the basic skills needed for nursing work in humanitarian settings?
- What are the five forms of self-care the author and his colleagues used to care for themselves while helping people suffering with Ebola?

    1.

    2.

    3.

    4.

    5.

why

Why is self-care even more important for humanitarian aid workers than traditional healthcare workers? What additional stressors do they face?

do

Activity 18-1: Fictional and Nonfictional Healthcare Workers

Read, or reread, a book about healthcare workers in challenging circumstances. We offer a few wonderful choices to get you started. As you read, consider how self-care factors into the subject's work, if at all.

The Plague, by Albert Camus

Cutting for Stone, by Abraham Verghese

The Shift, by Theresa Brown

Being Mortal, by Atul Gawande

Mountains Beyond Mountains, by Tracey Kidder

Activity 18-2: Interview Humanitarian or Pandemic Workers

Interview a student, a nurse peer, or a nursing professor who has worked in a humanitarian setting or during the AIDS epidemic of the 1980s and 1990s. You may also want to interview a nurse who worked during the COVID-19 pandemic. Ask them to describe the work they did and what motivated them to care for their patients. What challenges did they face? How did they take care of themselves? How did they balance their work with the concerns of their families and loved ones?

Activity 18-3: Blogging

We have encouraged you to reflect on your experiences with journal writing, but have you considered sharing your thoughts with others? Many humanitarian workers write online blogs so they can share their experience with others and feel heard, with the hope of creating change. Sharing personal narratives can be an opportunity for others, not only humanitarian nurses, to have their voices heard. Consider starting now. As a nursing student or early career nurse, what experiences would be of interest to others? What universal lessons and wisdom are you gaining that you could share with others? Determine your audience and your unique perspective, and write a blog post. You might also consider writing an editorial; your school of nursing probably has a communications director who would be willing to help you find a publication "home" for it.

reflect & journal

- This chapter reminds us that self-care must be fluid and flexible, not only in humanitarian settings but also in more traditional healthcare environments. When have you been successful in staying flexible during difficult situations? How did that flexibility benefit your well-being?

- Humor has been an important aspect of self-care for this author and others in humanitarian settings. But humor can be dark, and it can diminish those around us. This is especially fraught in healthcare settings. Have you experienced a time when you or others were using humor at other people's expense?

19
Sowing Seeds of Resilience: Compassionate Care Ambassadors

what

- Read Chapter 19.
- What is a Compassionate Care Ambassador?
- The Compassionate Care Ambassador program is just one example of nurses advocating to help other nurses. What are the steps the authors undertook to successfully launch their program?

why

Why is it so important for Ambassadors themselves to "walk the walk" of self-care and resilience?

do

Activity 19-1: Conduct a Needs Assessment

The foundation of the Compassionate Care Ambassador program described in this chapter was a needs assessment. Hospitals are not the only setting where people need well-being interventions. Schools of nursing are stressful, too. Conduct a needs assessment in your school. Use a focus group, survey, or discussion anywhere nursing students are gathered to identify students' priorities, challenges, and any unmet needs in your school. A word of caution: When we ask people what they need and then don't provide it, that lack of response can be frustrating. We encourage you to tell students that you are conducting this needs assessment as a class exercise so that expectations are clear. (Note, however, if you identify a need and would like to advocate for change, we will not argue with you on that! In fact, refer to Activity 19-2.)

Activity 19-2: Advocate for Change

In your needs assessment (Activity 19-1), you will identify changes that might significantly benefit the students at your school. These could range from extended hours for the coffee kiosk to a change in the grading system. Choose one change, probably something considered low-hanging fruit: a change that is simple and quick to implement, requiring few resources but potentially having a significant impact. How can you generate support for this change among school leadership? What outcomes would be linked to your proposed change? Be sure to frame the outcomes so that they reflect the goals of these leaders. (Longer coffee cart hours will increase students' ability to stay on campus longer, increasing study time and improving test scores. They also will foster increased socialization among students and faculty.) Is there any evidence in the research literature suggesting that these outcomes will be likely? Learn as much as you can about the costs and benefits of your proposed change. Write a one-page memo, and share it with the appropriate school leader. Schedule an appointment to discuss the change. Good luck!

Activity 19-3: Effective Change Agents

Think of someone you admire who has successfully fought for change. This person can be in healthcare, social justice, politics, or elsewhere. What qualities make this person an effective change agent? What skills do they have, and how do they use them effectively? What resources did they leverage to help them enable change?

reflect & journal

- We talk about advocating for change quite a bit in the textbook. This is, in part, because no work environment is perfect for all its patients or all its staff. There are many times when you will see the need for change, and each time, you must decide how you will respond. In some instances, fighting for change will be the best path. At other times, it might be best to leave that clinical setting for a place where the grass is truly greener. But as we said, no workplace is perfect. Learning to advocate for change, for yourself and others, will become an important skill.

- Think of a time you have successfully advocated for change, big or small.

- As you look around your school, your clinical site, and your community, what changes would you like to see? How can you play a role in addressing these changes?

section V
The Heart of a Nurse

20

Mattering: Creating a Rich Work Life

what

- Read Chapter 20.
- Mattering is a fascinating concept and one you probably haven't studied before. What are the four domains of interpersonal mattering?

    1.

    2.

    3.

    4.

- Explain the differences between interpersonal mattering and societal mattering.
- In the study conducted by the author, what were the opportunities for nurses to feel like they mattered at work?

why

- Why is mattering an important concept in the context of nursing education and training? Think not only of "traditional" nursing students, but students who tend to be marginalized.
- How does a sense of mattering factor into a nurse's sense of well-being and resilience?

do

Activity 20-1: When Do I Matter?

Take a moment to think about your experience as a nursing student. Who or what has made you feel like you matter? When have you felt seen or heard? How have you, or could you have, added value? Write or tell the story of a time when you felt like you mattered.

Activity 20-2: Mattering and Patient Care

Clinicals also provide an opportunity to spend a few extra minutes with a patient. What can you learn about that patient as a person? Perhaps they could share with you what their experience has been with the illness or issue that brought them to the hospital or clinic. How is this experience affecting their life? What do they value most about the care their nurses provide? What advice would they have for you as a future nurse? Asking questions and taking the time to listen to the answers provide a valuable service to anyone but is particularly important if a person is alone, confused, scared, or uncomfortable. You have the potential to make that person feel seen and heard and to show them that they matter. You can add value by helping that individual feel valued. You may also learn something that has been overlooked or not considered by the team caring for that person and can serve everyone involved by bringing that something to light.

Activity 20-3: Do Students Matter?

Clinical instructors and preceptors choose to work with student nurses because they are invested in your education. In addition to learning about physical assessment, medications, and the art of caring for another person, take a moment to learn something about your preceptor. Why did they choose nursing? What do they enjoy most about working with students? What is the most important thing they do in a day's work? Can your preceptor tell you about a time when they felt like they mattered? The answers to these questions will provide you with valuable insight into the profession of nursing and may provide a much-needed boost for your preceptor. We hope you will find that students play an important role in preceptors' sense of mattering.

reflect & journal

- The chapter ends by pointing out that there will be times you won't receive the feedback or recognition reminding you that you matter. What will you do to foster your own sense of mattering?

- How can you help others feel as if they matter? This can include fellow students, patients, and colleagues.

21
Integrating a Life That Works With a Life That Counts

what

- Read Chapter 21.
- Describe David Whyte's "three marriages" metaphor.

- List three ways to foster authenticity in your personal and work relationships.

  1.

  2.

  3.

- The chapter offers seven specific strategies for creating and maintaining an integrated life. What are they?

  1.

  2.

  3.

  4.

  5.

  6.

  7.

why

Why does the author prefer the term "work-life integration" over "work-life balance"?

do

Activity 21-1: Pebble in Your Shoe

The author talks about the Joy in Work project that revealed weekend and evening emails were a "pebble in the shoe" of her faculty. To increase joy in the workplace, the school simply stopped weekend and evening emails, as well as the expectation that these off-hours emails must be answered.

Consider a simple change you could make that could greatly improve your happiness and joy. Make that change, and see what happens when you no longer have that pebble in your shoe.

Activity 21-2: Eavesdropping

The first step in creating an integrated life is "knowing yourself" so that you will be free and able to reveal yourself to others. Give yourself time and space (at least 30 minutes) to imagine that it's your nursing school graduation celebration. All the most important people in your life are in attendance—family, friends, teachers, colleagues, patients, and more. You notice a group of them talking animatedly, smiling, and nodding. They are talking about how much they love and care about you and why. They share why they admire you, what they value most about you, and how you have had an impact on their lives. You overhear the entire conversation. What do they say?

reflect & journal

- In class, on the job, and at home, do you feel like you can fully be your authentic self? Are you living, studying, or working in a place where you find yourself coding your language or changing your actions to fit certain expectations? What keeps you from being authentic at times? Think about those expectations and their source. Now consider ways you can take steps to either share yourself more fully in these spaces or find spaces that are more supportive of your true self.

- Write a reflection on why you chose to become a nurse. Was it even a choice for you? We're guessing you've probably been asked this question a few times in nursing school, so this time, when you reflect on the "why" about your career choice, write about it in a way that gives you a sense of strength. What did you experience in your life that made you move in the direction of nursing? How did that experience make you better, stronger, and more knowledgeable about the world you live in? As you write, hang onto this journal entry and go back to it when times are tough in nursing school or your career. You can "bounce back" and remember where you came from, and use that as a source of strength and resilience.

22
Providing Compassionate Care and Addressing Unmet Social Needs Can Reduce Your Burnout

what

- Read Chapter 22.
- There are two kinds of compassionate care described in this chapter. What do we mean when we talk about "compassionate care"?
- Only 20% of patients' health outcomes are determined by the medical care they receive (University of Wisconsin Population Health Institute, 2014). List at least six nonmedical factors that affect a patient's health.

    1.

    2.

    3.

    4.

    5.

    6.

why

What are the benefits of compassionate care? Why is compassionate care such an important component of self-care?

do

Activity 22-1: Addressing Unmet Social Needs

Much has been written about social determinants of health, or the social factors that have a significant impact on patients' health. These include socioeconomic status, education, neighborhoods, employment, social support, and access to health care (Artiga & Hinton, 2018). This chapter describes some of the ways that nurses try to address these needs with food pantries as well as partnerships with social service agencies to connect patients with vital social services. How do your local hospitals identify and address these unmet social needs? How prevalent are these issues in your community? A lot of this information will be available through your local department of health and in agencies that address specific needs, such as mental health, substance use disorders, and maternal health.

Activity 22-2: Find Your Voice

In the final sidebar, Elizabeth Métraux advises: "You've found your calling, now find your voice—and your people." In this activity, we ask you to inventory your talents and skills that can become your voice as you advocate for your patients. Are you a good speaker? A compelling writer? A natural leader or persuader? When have you used these talents to effect change?

Activity 22-3: Find Your People

Next, find your people. Research advocacy groups at your institution and in your community. What issue are you especially passionate about? What are the national and international organizations that work to address this issue? Finally, learn about the advocacy work done by professional nursing and healthcare groups, such as the American Nurses Association or Partners in Health. Is there an organization that you would like to become a part of?

reflect & journal

- The chapter author shares her personal story of when her husband was in a fatal accident. What behaviors did his nurses, Abby and Kathy, exhibit that made such an impact on her? What impact did Abby and Kathy's compassionate care have on their own well-being?
- Métraux says it is "impossible to separate the well-being of providers from the pain endured by patients." How does it feel to know that your own well-being is woven into the well-being of those around you, especially those who may be suffering deeply? What implications does this have for you?

references

Artiga, S., & Hinton, E. (2018, May). Beyond health care: The role of social determinants in promoting health and health equity (Issue Brief). Henry J. Kaiser Family Foundation. https://www.kff.org/disparities-policy/issue-brief/beyond-health-care-the-role-of-social-determinants-in-promoting-health-and-health-equity/

University of Wisconsin Population Health Institute. (2014). *County health rankings key findings.* Robert Wood Johnson Foundation. https://www.countyhealthrankings.org/sites/default/files/2014%20County%20Health%20Rankings%20Key%20Findings.pdf

23

Showing Up With Grit and Grace: How to Lead Under Pressure as a Nurse Clinician and Leader

what

- Read Chapter 23.
- How would you define *grit*? (You may also want to refer to Chapter 2.) How does Manny exhibit grit in this chapter? Provide two examples of grit that you have practiced or witnessed as a nursing student.
- How would you define *grace*? How does Manny exhibit grace? List two examples of grace that you have practiced or witnessed as a nursing student.
- What does the author mean by the term *leading mindfully*?

why

Why are grit and grace such important foundations for effective leaders? Please keep in mind that *everyone* is a leader, not just those at the top of the organizational charts.

do

Activity 23-1: Resilience Map

Do the same exercise that Manny did, mapping his resilience on a typical day. As you recall, he woke up tired and sluggish, went through stages of hyperarousal during work, crashed and felt irritated and exhausted toward the end of his shift, and came home with no energy left at all. Map your resilience using the example in Figure 23.4. Narrate your map. What do you notice? Are there small changes you can try with the goal of maximizing your time spent in the resilient zone?

Activity 23-2: Wrappers on the Cart

We love that Manny's story epitomizes what so many authors have shared in the textbook, including both the art of reframing and the power of perspective. Manny discovered that he had the capacity to *choose* how he perceived those wrappers on the carts each morning. The circumstance—wrappers on the carts—was always the same, but Manny's thoughts about them changed. Initially he was annoyed and irritated by them. They made him feel unappreciated and put upon. When he changed his thoughts to see the wrappers as reminders that his colleagues, too, were busy and overworked, his thoughts about the wrappers—and his colleagues—changed. He felt compassion toward his coworkers, and one result of this change was Manny's own well-being.

Do you have a pet peeve? What regularly annoys you? Reframe your personal "wrappers on the cart" and see what happens. You have the power to choose.

Activity 23-3: Arrive-Breathe-Connect

Follow the instructions for the Arrive-Breathe-Connect exercise in Chapter 23. For the next week, practice this exercise at least once a day. Which is easier for you to connect to: grit or grace?

reflect & journal

The chapter author writes that "while you perform, you are also leading, because others are consciously and unconsciously picking up on your cues. Whether or not you and others are aware of it, how you show up in the moment leads others through the power of *your* example." We don't always realize how much power we have in any given situation. We have the ability to turn everything around simply by our presence, demeanor, and grace. In the coming week, pay attention to your own power to influence those around you, hopefully in a positive way!